UNLOCKING

THE

PUZZLE

Navigating the Complexities of Autism

Dr. Macklene. C. Jones

CONTENTS

Introduction

"Unlocking the Puzzle: Navigating Autism's Complexities." This book is a thorough reference that sheds light on the complex and multidimensional world of autism. This book seeks to provide you with a deeper understanding and practical insights regarding autism, whether you are a parent, caregiver, educator, or simply inquisitive about this neurological disorder.

Autism, often known as autism spectrum disorder (ASD), is a neurological disorder that affects millions of people worldwide. Its various forms, ranging from difficulties with social interaction and communication to restricted interests and repetitive behaviors, can provide distinct problems for persons with autism and their families. With the rising prevalence of autism diagnoses, there is an urgent need to untangle the complexity behind the disorder. In this book, we set out to solve the mysteries of autism, investigating its origins, the elements that contribute to its development, and the impact it has on people's lives. We will look at scientific studies, share personal tales, and offer practical techniques for overcoming problems and enjoying the qualities of those on the autism spectrum.

We will piece together the jigsaw of autism chapter by chapter, beginning with a detailed investigation of what autism truly is. We will look at the historical context and changing opinions on autism, highlighting the various manifestations. Understanding the entire spectrum is critical for appreciating the distinct experiences and needs of people on various spectrums.

Following that, we shall investigate the underlying causes of autism. We will look at recent research and findings that offer insight into the neurological underpinnings of autism, from genetic factors to environmental triggers. By putting these puzzle pieces together, we hope to create a more complete picture of the condition's beginnings and develop a better understanding of its intricacies.

Finally, we will discuss the practical aspects of overcoming the problems of autism. For early intervention and assistance, early detection and diagnosis are critical. Communication difficulties and techniques will be investigated, allowing people with autism to express themselves and interact with others more successfully. We will also look into a variety of supportive interventions and therapies that help improve quality of life and general well-being. We hope that this book will develop empathy, understanding, and acceptance of people with autism. Our objective is to give you useful information, practical solutions, and resources to help you negotiate the complexity of autism with confidence and compassion.

So, let us go on this adventure together, solving the autism puzzle and celebrating the extraordinary potential and unique perspectives of those on the autism spectrum.

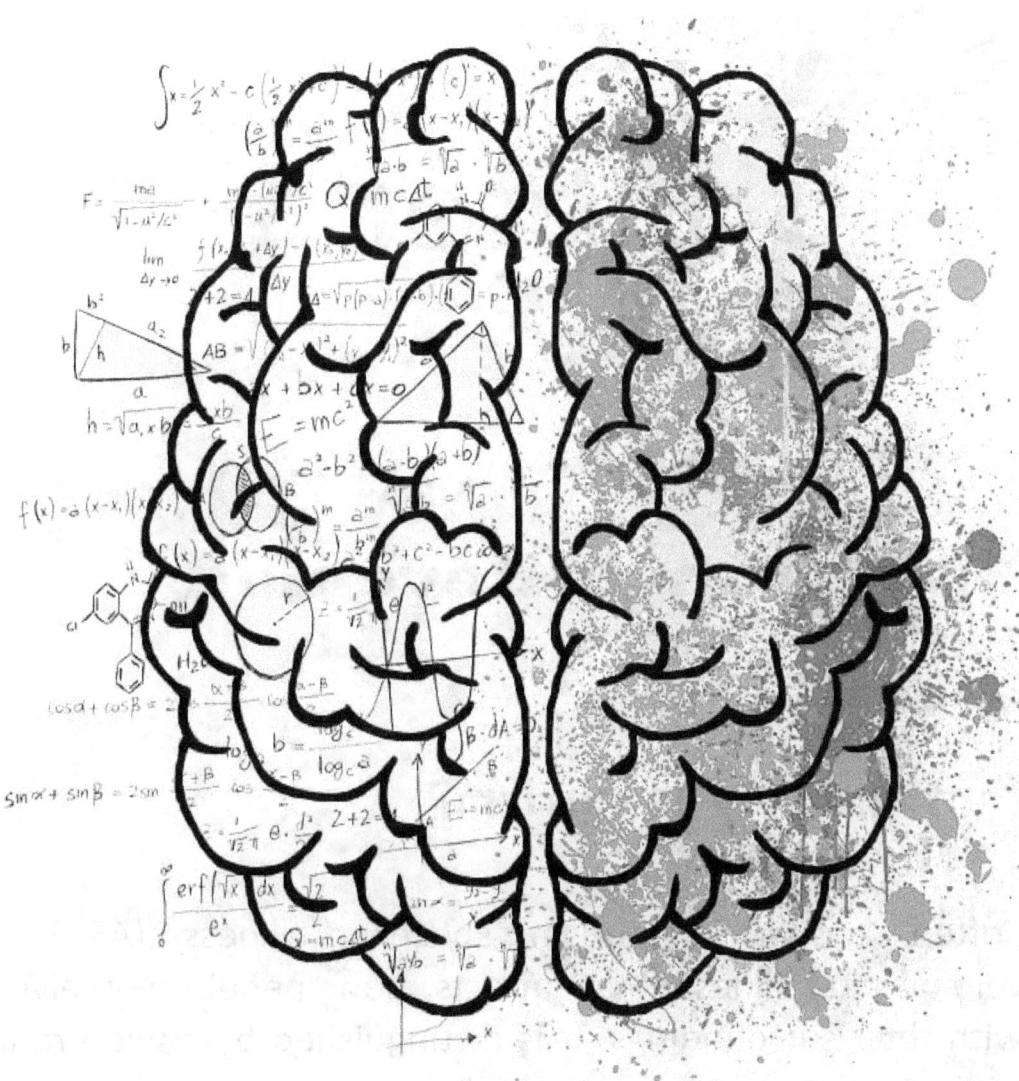

Chapter 1

The Spectrum is Revealed

1.1 What exactly is autism?

Autism, often known as autism spectrum illness (ASD), is a neurodevelopmental illness that affects how people perceive and interact with their surroundings. It is distinguished by a wide range of difficulties in social communication and engagement, as well as constrained and repetitive patterns of behavior, hobbies, or activities.

One of the hallmarks of autism is difficulty with social contact. Individuals with autism may have difficulty interpreting and responding to social cues, making it difficult for them to engage in ordinary social interactions. They may struggle to read nonverbal signs such as facial expressions, tone of voice, and body language, which can impair their understanding of others' intentions and feelings. As a result, autistic people may struggle to build and sustain relationships, and they may prefer solitary pursuits to social engagements.

Autism also has a significant impact on communication. Some people with autism may have delays in speech and language development, while others may struggle with pragmatic language skills. Comprehending and using language in social circumstances, such as taking turns in conversation, using proper body language, and comprehending sarcasm or comedy, is part of pragmatic language. These issues might cause misunderstandings and make good communication difficult.

Autism patients frequently demonstrate confined and repetitive patterns of behavior, hobbies, or activities. They may exhibit repetitive motions or activities such as hand flapping, rocking, or object lining. They may also exhibit extreme fixations on specific themes or objects and deep understanding and enthusiasm in those particular subjects. Furthermore, people with autism frequently rely on routine and predictability, and changes from familiar routines can create difficulty or worry.

It's critical to remember that autism is a spectrum disorder. The term "spectrum" refers to the vast range of abilities, strengths, and challenges that people with autism display. Some people may require extensive assistance in their daily lives, but others may be quite independent and excel in specialized areas. The spectrum viewpoint recognizes the individuality of each person's experiences and highlights the significance of adapting assistance and treatments to match their distinct needs.

Understanding autism entails understanding and respecting the various ways it manifests. We can learn more about autism by studying its key characteristics, and increase understanding, acceptance, and support for people on the autism spectrum. Throughout this book, we will investigate the complexities of autism, to provide a complete understanding as well as practical solutions for navigating its hurdles and realizing its incredible potential.

1.2 Autism's Historical Perspectives

Autism's understanding and recognition have evolved greatly over time. Exploring historical perspectives on autism offers useful insights into how our understanding and perception of this neurodevelopmental condition have evolved.

Autism-like observations were first observed in the early twentieth century. However, it wasn't until the mid-twentieth century that autism was recognized as a unique condition. Dr. Leo Kanner, an Austrian-American psychiatrist, was a pivotal player in the history of autism. Dr. Kanner produced a seminal paper in 1943 that coined the term "infantile autism" and identified a group of children with social and communication difficulties, limited interests, and repetitive habits. His observations were a watershed moment in the history of autism and were among the first systematic efforts to describe and characterize the illness.

At the same time, another researcher, Hans Asperger, was investigating a group of children with similar features on his own. Asperger's work shed light on a new aspect of the autism spectrum, eventually dubbed Asperger's Syndrome. While Dr. Kanner focused on people with more severe disabilities, Asperger emphasized the unique abilities and characteristics displayed by people on the autism spectrum.

Autism research progressed in the decades that followed, resulting in increased awareness and the improvement of diagnostic criteria. Significant adjustments to the diagnostic criteria occurred, with the introduction of larger categories such as "pervasive developmental disorders" and finally consolidation under the umbrella term "autism spectrum disorder" (ASD) in the Diagnostic and Statistical Manual of Mental Disorders (DSM).

As social knowledge developed, attempts were made to dispel myths and question widely held beliefs regarding the causes of autism. Misguided notions in the past attributed autism to variables such as "refrigerator mothers" or parental behavior. These theories have been widely debunked, and our understanding of autism has turned toward recognizing the intricate interplay of genetic, environmental, and neurological variables in its development.

The late-twentieth-century development of the neurodiversity movement was critical in altering attitudes toward autism. This movement advocates for the acceptance and celebration of neurological impairments, such as autism, as a natural component of human diversity. It promotes inclusiveness, self-advocacy, and valuing the strengths and unique perspectives of those on the autism spectrum.

Today, we have a better understanding of autism. Continues to evolve as a result of continuous brain research and advancements. With a broader perspective, we see that autism is not a defect that must be corrected, but rather a difference that must be understood and supported. Autism's historical perspectives have led the way for increased understanding, acceptance, and the development of effective interventions and support techniques for people with autism and their families.

We may better comprehend the problems experienced by earlier generations and pave the road for a more inclusive and enlightened future by appreciating the historical background and the journey of knowledge surrounding autism.

1.3   Recognizing   Autism's   Variable Presentations

As a spectrum disorder, autism comprises a wide range of presentations and manifestations. Recognizing and comprehending the various ways in which autism manifests itself is critical for acknowledging the distinct experiences and needs of people on the spectrum.

The variety in social communication and interaction abilities is one of the fundamental elements of autism's various presentations. While some people with autism have substantial issues recognizing and responding to social cues, others may have more subtle impairments that go unreported. Some people have great verbal talents but suffer from pragmatic language use in social circumstances, whilst others have limited speech and rely on alternative modes of communication such as gestures, signs, or assistive technology. The existence of restricted and repetitive activities and interests is another element of autism's various manifestations. While repetitive motions and behaviors are frequently linked to autism, they can appear in a variety of ways. Some people may engage in repeated or stereotyped movements such as hand flapping, spinning, or rocking. Others may become obsessed with specific topics or objects, displaying great knowledge and proficiency in those areas. Furthermore, devotion to routines and aversion to change is frequent qualities among people with autism, albeit the amount of these characteristics varies.

Sensory processing abnormalities are another important feature of autism's various manifestations. Autistic people may have increased or decreased sensitivity to sensory stimuli such as sounds, lighting, textures, tastes, or odors. This can result in Sensory overload or sensory-seeking behavior. Individuals with autism may experience sensory impairments in a variety of ways, affecting their comfort and ability to manage their environments efficiently.

Furthermore, the level of support required varies greatly across the autism spectrum. Some people may require considerable assistance in their daily life, such as with self-care, communicating, and controlling sensory sensitivities. Others may be extremely self-sufficient and possess exceptional talents and strengths in specialized areas such as mathematics, music, art, or problem-solving. Recognizing and accepting this spectrum of abilities and support needs is critical for delivering appropriate treatments and promoting individual growth and well-being.

By acknowledging the various manifestations of autism, we may move beyond stereotypes and recognize that each person's experience is unique. It enables us to recognize and solve the issues that people with autism may confront while also appreciating their amazing skills and talents. Accepting neurodiversity and encouraging inclusive environments that meet the different needs of people on the autism spectrum are critical steps toward creating a society that values and supports the full range of human experiences.

How to Handle Autistic Outbursts and Difficulties

Coping with autism outbursts and difficult times can be difficult, but with understanding, patience, and appropriate solutions, these situations can be navigated more effectively. Here are some coping strategies for autistic outbursts and challenging times:

Maintain cool: It is critical to maintain your cool through eruptions or difficult times. By being calm, you can contribute to the individual's sense of stability and security. Take deep breaths, employ calming techniques, and keep in mind that your reaction has an impact on the circumstance.

Create Predictability and Routine: To reduce anxiety and potential triggers, create a structured and predictable atmosphere.

15

Set up consistent routines and schedules, with visual aids and explicit expectations. Predictability and routine can be beneficial in assisting individuals with autism to feel safer and lessen the probability of outbursts.

Recognize Triggers: Be aware of patterns and triggers that lead to outbursts or tough moments. Observe and record any environmental, sensory, or social elements that appear to provoke unpleasant responses. You can reduce the chance of outbursts by identifying triggers and working to avoid or minimize them.

Use Visual Supports and Social Stories: Visual supports, such as visual timetables, social stories, and visual signals, can help people with autism prepare for difficult circumstances. To express expectations, steps, or changes in routines, use visual supports. Individuals can use social stories to understand and cope with tough emotions or transitions.

Encourage Communication and Self-Expression: Encourage individuals with autism to express themselves through open lines of communicating their emotions and needs. Alternative communication modalities, such as visual assistance, sign language, or augmentative and alternative communication (AAC) devices, should be made available. Validate their emotions and sentiments by assisting them in finding suitable methods to express themselves.

Provide Sensory Support: Sensory sensitivity might contribute to outbursts or difficult moments. Determine sensory preferences and sensitivities and offer the necessary help. Offering sensory breaks, providing sensory tools or fidget toys, or creating a sensory-friendly atmosphere with less sensory stimulation are all examples of this.

Teach Coping techniques: Assist people with autism in developing and practicing coping techniques to help them regulate their emotions and reactions. Deep breathing exercises, relaxing techniques, self-regulation measures, or diverting attention to different hobbies or interests are all examples. Work with therapists or other specialists to develop appropriate coping methods.

Seek Professional Help: If the outbursts or difficult periods continue and have a substantial impact on everyday functioning, consider obtaining professional help. Occupational therapists, behavior analyzers, and psychologists who specialize in autism can offer valuable insights, methods, and interventions for addressing problematic behaviors and promoting emotional well-being.

Caregivers must take care of their well-being when dealing with autism outbursts and difficult times. Maintain support systems and engage in self-care activities that help you relax, rejuvenate, and manage stress. Seek help from friends, relatives, or support groups who can relate to your situation.

Remember that each autistic person is unique, and what works for one person may not work for another. It is critical to be adaptive and flexible, always learning and altering techniques dependent on the situation and individual's needs and preferences. You may negotiate and cope with autism outbursts and difficult moments more effectively if you have empathy, understanding, and a supportive approach.

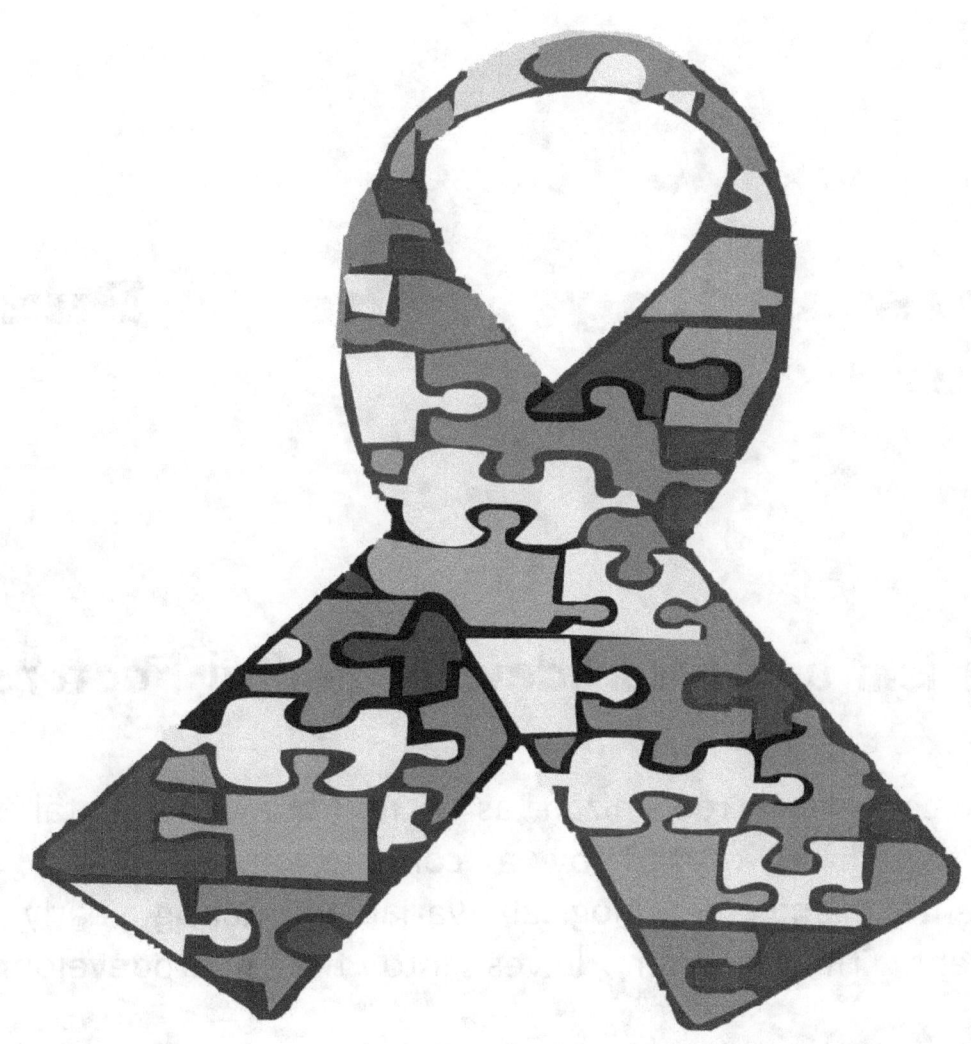

Chapter 2

Understanding the Puzzle Pieces

2.1 Autism and Neurodevelopmental Factors

Autism is commonly recognized as a neurodevelopmental illness, implying that it is caused by a complex interplay of genetic, environmental, and neurological variables during early brain development. This chapter delves into the neurodevelopmental variables linked to autism, examining the many puzzle pieces that lead to its emergence.

2.1.1 Genetic Factors

Autism has a major hereditary component, according to research. Certain genetic variants and mutations have been shown in studies to enhance the likelihood of developing autism. While the specific genes involved and their interactions are still being studied, it is obvious that numerous genes have a role in autism development. These genetic variables contribute to the condition's underlying neurobiology, altering brain development, brain connections, and critical neurotransmitter function.

2.1.2 Triggers in the Environment

While genetics play a part, environmental variables also play a role in the development of autism. Several environmental variables during pregnancy and early childhood have been studied for their potential link to autism. Prenatal infections, exposure to specific drugs, and maternal immune system activation have all been investigated as potential risk factors. Furthermore, prenatal and early postnatal exposure to environmental toxins, such as air pollution and certain chemicals, has been linked to an increased risk of autism. It is crucial to emphasize that while environmental influences are unlikely to cause autism on their own, they may interact with a genetic predisposition to contribute to its development.

2.1.3 Brain Growth and Connectivity

The brain is crucial. Studies have found anatomical and functional differences in the brains of people with autism compared to neurotypical people. Neuronal proliferation, migration, and synaptic pruning are processes that shape the complicated neural networks throughout early brain development. Disruptions in these systems can have an impact on brain connections and result in the abnormal neural activity patterns seen in autism. Contributing elements have been identified as changes in brain areas involved in social cognition, communication, and sensory processing.

2.1.4 Imbalance in Excitation-Inhibition

A mismatch in the stimulation and inhibition of brain activity is another neurodevelopmental component linked to autism. The brain's delicate balance of excitatory and inhibitory messages is critical for appropriate functioning. According to research, people with autism may have an imbalance favoring excitement over inhibition, which can impact information processing, sensory integration, and neuronal network control. This mismatch contributes to the unusual patterns of brain activity seen in autistic people.

Understanding the neurodevelopmental aspects related to autism provides vital insights into the condition's underlying mechanisms. It emphasizes the intricate interplay of genetic and environmental effects, as well as the impact on brain growth and connectivity. By putting these puzzle pieces together, we may gain a better understanding of autism and set the framework for designing customized therapies and support measures that address the specific neurological elements in action.

2.2 Autism Genetic Influences

Autism development is heavily influenced by genetic factors. Extensive research has revealed that certain genetic variants and mutations increase the likelihood of acquiring autism spectrum disorder (ASD). This section delves into the genetic factors linked to autism and their impact on the progression of this complicated neurodevelopmental disorder.

2.2.1 Autism's Polygenic Nature

Autism is classified as a polygenic condition, which means that it is caused by the interplay of numerous genes. Numerous genes have been linked to autism, and the specific roles and interactions of these genes are still being studied. These genes are engaged in a variety of biological processes that are essential for brain development, neuronal connection, and neurotransmitter function.

2.2.2 Rare genetic variants and copy number variations

Some people who have autistic patients have rare genetic abnormalities or mutations that enhance their likelihood of developing the disorder greatly. Chromosome abnormalities, such as copy number variants (CNVs), in which regions of DNA are duplicated or deleted, are examples of these changes. Certain CNVs, such as chromosomal duplications or deletions of certain areas, have been linked to an elevated risk of autism.

2.2.3 Typical Genetic Variations

Common genetic variants, in addition to unusual genetic changes, contribute to the risk of autism. These polymorphisms are more common in the general population, but they nevertheless have an impact on the development of the illness. Several common genetic variations have been linked to an elevated risk of autism in genome-wide association studies (GWAS). It is crucial to note, however, that each of these frequent variations confers it is only a minor danger, but the combined effect of several variations is significant.

2.2.4 Interactions Between Genes and Environment

Autism genetic variables do not function in isolation but can interact with environmental factors to cause the condition to develop. The interaction between genetic susceptibility and environmental stimuli has been studied. Certain genetic differences, for example, may enhance vulnerability to environmental influences such as prenatal infections, activation of the mother's immune system, or exposure to environmental pollutants. Understanding these gene-environment interactions can give light on how genetic predisposition and environmental effects contribute to autism development.

2.2.5 Heterogeneity in Genetics

Autism is marked by considerable genetic heterogeneity, which means that distinct genetic variations and combinations can result in clinical symptoms and diagnoses that are comparable. This genetic diversity contributes to the varied presentations and phenotypic heterogeneity observed in people with autism. It also emphasizes the complexities of the autism genetic landscape and the difficulties in identifying exact genetic markers or particular causal genes.

The study of autism's hereditary impacts provides critical insights into the condition's basic origins. It contributes to a better understanding of the complex connections between genes, their involvement in brain development and connectivity, and their susceptibility to environmental variables. We can pave the path for early detection, personalized therapies, and targeted support measures suited to the distinct genetic profiles of individuals with autism by unraveling the genetic puzzle pieces of autism.

2.3 Autism and Environmental Triggers

While genetics is important in the development of autism, environmental variables significantly influence the risk and manifestation of autism spectrum disorder (ASD). In this section, we look at the environmental triggers that have been researched about autism, as well as their possible impact on the development of this complicated neurological condition.

2.3.1 Risk Factors During Pregnancy

Prenatal variables have been intensively researched for their potential link to autism. As putative environmental causes, several prenatal disorders and events have been investigated:

Maternal illnesses during pregnancy, such as rubella, cytomegalovirus (CMV), and influenza, have been linked to an increased risk of autism. The immune response triggered by these illnesses may have an impact on embryonic brain development, resulting in neural changes in circuits, as well as an elevated risk of acquiring autism.

2.3.1.2 Maternal Immune System Activation

During pregnancy, activation of the maternal immune system, such as in reaction to infections or autoimmune illnesses, has been associated with an increased risk of autism in offspring. The immune response and the related release of inflammatory chemicals are thought to alter embryonic brain development, resulting in long-term abnormalities in neural functioning.

2.3.1.3 Medications and Substances

specific medications, such as valproic acid (an anticonvulsant) and thalidomide (used to treat specific disorders), have been linked to an elevated risk of autism when used during pregnancy. Furthermore, exposure to certain chemicals during pregnancy, such as alcohol and smoke, has been associated with an increased risk.

2.3.2 Factors Influencing Early Childhood Development

Environmental early childhood triggers have also been studied for their potential impact on autism risk:

Air Pollution: Early childhood exposure to air pollution has been related to an increased risk of autism. Fine particulate matter and traffic-related contaminants may have neurotoxic effects, affecting brain development and contributing to the development of autism.

Maternal Stress: Maternal stress during pregnancy and early childhood has been explored as a potential environmental cause for autism. Chronic maternal stress, such as anxiety or depression, may have an impact on fetal brain development and contribute to an increased risk of autism.

Parental Age: Both maternal and paternal advanced parental age have been linked to an increased risk of autism. The precise processes underlying this relationship are not entirely known, although they may involve a higher likelihood of genetic mutations or changes in gene epigenetic control.

It is vital to emphasize that environmental factors are unlikely to induce autism on their own. They are thought to interact with genetic predispositions and other variables, contributing to the condition's risk and manifestation. The interaction of genetic vulnerability and environmental effects is still being studied.

Understanding the probable environmental triggers associated with autism helps us better understand the complicated elements that contribute to its development. It emphasizes the relevance of prenatal and early childhood circumstances in determining neural development and emphasizes the necessity for pregnant women and young children to be in supportive, healthy situations. Recognizing can reduce the influence of environmental factors that may contribute to autism risk by addressing them and encouraging optimal neurodevelopment for all children.

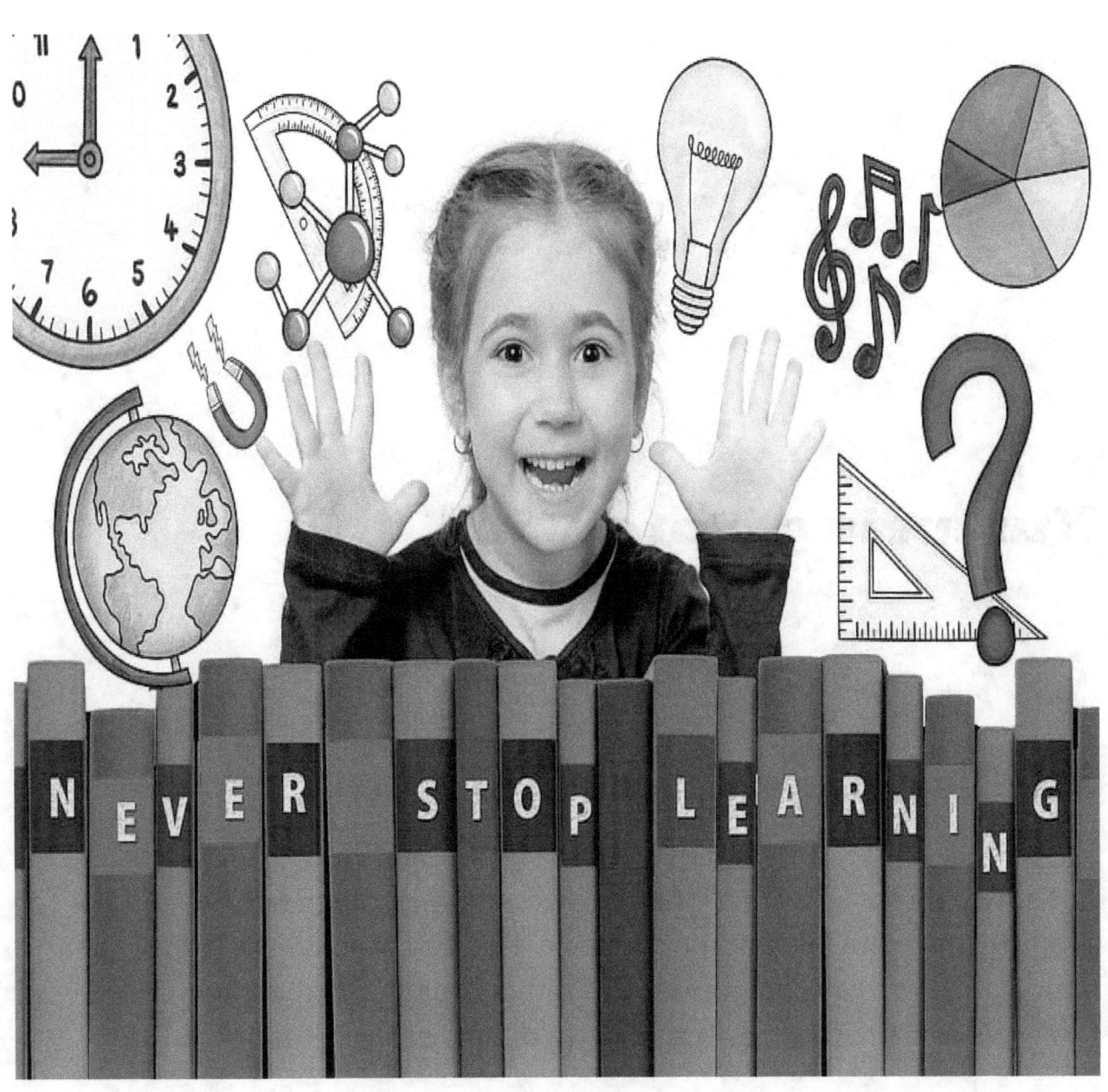

Chapter 3

Nurturing Potential

3.1 Diagnosis and Early Detection

Autism spectrum disorder (ASD) screening and diagnosis are critical for prompt intervention and support. In this chapter, we will look at the importance of early diagnosis, the difficulties in diagnosing autism, and the tools and procedures that can help with early detection.

3.1.1 The Value of Early Detection

Early autism discovery allows for early intervention, which can have a substantial impact on a child's development and outcomes. Early intervention has been proven in studies to increase communication skills, social interactions, adaptive behaviors, and cognitive functioning in children with autism. Early detection of autism allows for access to appropriate services, therapies, and educational support suited to the individual's needs, maximizing the individual's potential for growth and development.

3.1.2 Obstacles in Autism Diagnosis

An autism diagnosis can be difficult because it is based on seeing and assessing behavioral traits. The variety in symptom presentation and overlap with other developmental problems can make a correct diagnosis difficult. Furthermore, young children may exhibit developmental differences that are transient or related to other factors, making it difficult to distinguish between typical and atypical development associated with autism. Delays in diagnosis can also be caused by cultural and linguistic factors, as well as differences in healthcare access and awareness.

3.1.3 Screening and Assessment Tools

Screening tools are used to identify children who may be at risk for autism and warrant further assessment. Widely used screening tools include the Modified Checklist for Autism in Toddlers (M-CHAT) and the

Social Communication SCQ, which stands for structured questionnaire. Parent-reported questionnaires are used in these instruments to assess several domains of development, including social communication skills, repetitive behaviors, and sensory sensitivity.

Comprehensive diagnostic exams include interdisciplinary evaluations conducted by professionals with autism diagnosis experience. Direct observation, planned play-based evaluations, and standardized testing that measure several elements of development, like communication, social interaction, and behavior, are common.

3.1.4 The Importance of Interdisciplinarity

A multidisciplinary approach comprising professionals from several professions, like psychologists, speech-language pathologists, developmental pediatricians, and occupational therapists, is required for accurate and fast autism diagnosis. Collaboration among these professionals ensures a thorough examination that takes into account all elements of development and provides a holistic knowledge of the child's strengths and weaknesses.

3.1.5 Early Intervention and Assistance

Once a diagnosis has been made, early intervention services are critical in assisting autistic children and their families. Early intervention programs may include ABA, speech therapy, occupational therapy, social skills training, and parent education. These therapies are targeted to the child's specific needs and aim to promote social communication, language development, adaptive abilities, and behavioral difficulties.

Efforts have been undertaken in recent years to raise autism awareness and improve early detection. Healthcare practitioners, schools, and parents are encouraged to keep a close eye on developmental milestones and to seek professional help if they have any concerns. We can improve early identification and diagnosis by raising awareness, increasing access to screening technologies, fostering effective teamwork among specialists, ensuring that children with autism receive the care they require at the earliest possible stage, and setting them on a path of optimal development and well-being.

3.2 Communication Problems and Solutions

Autism spectrum disorder (ASD) is distinguished by communication impairments. In this section, we look at the communication issues that people with autism encounter, as well as strategies and interventions for improving their communication skills and creating meaningful connections.

3.2.1 Language and Communication Development

Many people with autism have delays or differences in their language and speech development. Some people struggle to learn spoken language, while others exhibit echolalia (repetitive echoing of words or phrases) or idiosyncratic language (using unique phrases or words).

Communication problems can impair both expressive language (verbal output) and receptive language (understanding spoken language), making it challenging for individuals with autism to properly articulate their views and understand others.

3.2.2 Nonverbal Communication

Individuals with autism face substantial difficulty when it comes to body language, facial expressions, and gestures. Difficulties in reading and employing nonverbal signs can disrupt social interactions and impede the formation of meaningful relationships. Individuals with autism may fail to establish eye contact, understand social nuances, and interpret subtle signs, resulting in social communication issues.

3.2.3 AAC (Augmentative and Alternate Communication)

Individuals with limited verbal ability or those who are nonverbal can benefit from augmentative and alternative communication (AAC) technologies to express their thoughts and needs. AAC methods include using picture-based communication boards, sign language, technological devices with speech output, and communication applications. These tools and tactics can help autistic people communicate successfully and participate in meaningful activities.

3.2.4 Pragmatic Language and Social Communication

Pragmatic language refers to the social components of communication, such as taking turns, initiating and maintaining dialogues, understanding social signs, and modifying communication style depending on the situation. Individuals with autism frequently suffer from pragmatic language abilities, which can interfere with their ability to engage in reciprocal discussions and successfully manage social interactions. Individuals with autism can benefit from targeted therapies such as social skills training and structured play activities, which can help them build pragmatic language skills and improve their social communication abilities.

3.2.5 Supportive Visuals and Structured Communication

Visual supports, such as visual schedules, social stories, and visual clues, can help people with autism improve their communication and comprehension skills. Visual supports depict information, routines, and expectations visually, supporting individuals with autism in understanding and managing their regular routines. These aids can help to reduce anxiety, increase predictability, and improve communication and understanding.

3.2.6 Person-Centered and Individualized Approaches

Recognizing that communication patterns vary greatly among people with autism, it is critical to use personalized strategies.

Proven strategies for improving an autistic child's academic performance

Improving academic performance for people with autism necessitates a multifaceted strategy that takes into account their specific talents, problems, and learning styles. While every person is unique, some tried-and-true tactics and approaches can help with academic growth and achievement. Here are some helpful strategies for improving academic performance in people with autism:

Individualized Education Plan (IEP): Work with educators, therapists, and parents to create an IEP that defines precise academic goals, adjustments, and support services suited to the requirements of the individual. An IEP guarantees that students receive specialized attention and targeted interventions to help them succeed in school.

Structured and Visual Supports: Use visual aids, schedules, and organizational tools to improve comprehension and provide a predictable learning environment. Visual supports might include visual timetables, visual clues, and visual aids. Individuals with autism benefit from social stories and visual organizers to help them understand instructions, routines, and expectations.

Clear and plain Instruction: Break academic activities down into smaller, more doable steps, and provide clear and plain directions. To improve comprehension, use visual presentations, hands-on exercises, and concrete examples. Allow for plenty of practice and reinforcement of abilities.

Multisensory Approaches: To improve understanding and retention, use several senses in the learning process. Lessons should include visual, aural, tactile, and kinesthetic aspects. To reinforce topics, for example, employ manipulatives, films, interactive software, and movement-based exercises. Provide specific training and opportunity for the development of social skills. To address social communication, perspective-taking, and collaborative learning, work with speech-language pathologists or social skills trainers. Social skills training can improve peer interactions, group work, and communication as well as general academic involvement.

Positive Reinforcement: Use a positive reinforcement strategy to inspire and reward academic accomplishments and efforts. Determine meaningful rewards that are significant to the individual, such as favorite activities, tokens, or privileges. Celebrate accomplishments to enhance self-esteem and create a good learning atmosphere.

Exploration and implementation of relevant assistive technology tools to support learning and academic work. Speech-to-text software, text-to-speech tools, visual organizers, calculators, and educational apps created for people with special needs are examples of this.

Collaboration and communication: Encourage open lines of communication among parents, educators, therapists, and support personnel. Exchange information, progress reports, and strategies regularly to guarantee a consistent and coordinated approach across all environments. Effective academic support can result from collaborative problem-solving.

Sensory Interruptions and Self-Regulation: Recognize how sensory sensitivities affect academic performance. Allow them regular sensory breaks and self-regulation opportunities to maintain focus and attention. Include sensory-friendly tactics such as sensory gadgets, quiet areas, and movement breaks.

Peer Support and Inclusion: Promote peer support, social inclusion, and collaborative opportunities in academic environments. Encourage peer understanding, empathy, and acceptance to foster a friendly and inclusive learning environment.

Remember that each autistic person is unique, and what works for one person may not work for another. It is critical to observe, listen, and change techniques based on the responses and preferences of the individual. Individuals with autism can thrive academically and attain their full potential by using individualized and evidence-based techniques.

Art and Autism

Autism and art have a distinct and frequently entangled relationship. Many people on the autistic spectrum have extraordinary artistic ability and a strong interest and talent in a variety of art forms. Individuals with autism can communicate, explore their feelings, and share their unique viewpoints with the world through artistic expression.

Art and autism are amazing in the way it surpasses typical ways of communication. Individuals with autism can express themselves, convey their views, and communicate their experiences through art, even when verbal communication is difficult. Individuals with autism can express their feelings, thoughts, and fantasies in ways that others can understand through visual arts, music, dance, theater, and other creative avenues.

Art also provides individuals with autism a means to explore and understand the world around them. Many people on the autism spectrum have a keen sense of detail, a distinct way of perceiving their surroundings, and a deep obsession with patterns and repetition. These attributes are frequently seen in their artistic works, where meticulous details, precision, and repeated patterns can be seen. Individuals with autism use art to comprehend and make sense of their circumstances, as well as to communicate their worldview.

Furthermore, engaging in artistic endeavors can be quite helpful for those with autism. Art provides a nonjudgmental and encouraging environment for self-expression, self-discovery, and self-confidence development. It can be used to facilitate emotional discharge, stress reduction, and sensory integration. Art therapy, in particular, uses the creative process and artistic materials to help people explore their emotions, improve social skills, boost self-esteem, and promote general well-being.

Individuals with autism benefit from art in ways other than personal expression and therapeutic advantages. Their distinct aesthetic perspectives add to the art world's richness and enrichment. Autism-related artwork frequently offers a distinctness, uniqueness, and fresh perspective that captivates audiences. The art community has increasingly recognized and celebrated the abilities and achievements of autistic artists, developing forums and exhibitions dedicated to presenting their work.

Art can also help to raise awareness and understanding of autism. Individuals with autism can communicate through their artistic endeavors. Break down barriers and foster autism discourse by challenging preconceptions. Their artwork is an effective advocacy tool, demonstrating the potential, inventiveness, and unique viewpoints of those on the autistic spectrum.

To summarize, the relationship between autism and art is broad and multifaceted. Art allows autistic people to express themselves, communicate, explore, and receive therapy. It enables people to share their unique insights, enrich the art world, and boost autism awareness. We create opportunities for individuals with autism to have their voices heard, their abilities acknowledged, and their contributions recognized and respected by embracing and cultivating their artistic talents.

3.3 Interventions and Therapies for Support

Individuals with autism spectrum disorder (ASD) benefit greatly from supportive interventions and therapies that promote their well-being and development. In this section, we will look at various interventions and therapies that are effective in addressing the unique issues that people with autism encounter.

3.3.1 AB A (Applied Behavior Analysis)

Applied Behavior Analysis (ABA) is a well-known and evidence-based technique for autistic people. ABA focuses on recognizing and changing behaviors by breaking them down into smaller components and using methodical strategies to encourage desired behaviors while decreasing problematic ones. Individualized ABA interventions may involve discrete trial teaching, naturalistic teaching methodologies, and behavior management techniques. ABA aims to improve functional skills, independence, and social interactions while minimizing problematic behaviors.

3.3.2 Speech and Language Therapy

Speech and language therapy is a critical intervention for people who struggle with communication. SLPs help people with autism to improve their speech production, language comprehension, and expressive language skills. Therapy sessions may concentrate on articulation, vocabulary expansion, grammar development, pragmatic language skills enhancement, and social communication facilitation. To help with communication, augmentative and alternative communication (AAC) systems can be used.

3.3.3 Occupational Therapy

Occupational therapy (OT) attempts to improve people's independence and engagement in daily activities. OT therapies for autistic people may focus on fine and gross motor abilities, sensory processing and control, self-care skills, and promoting adaptive behaviors. Sensory integration strategies and motor coordination may be used in OT sessions, activities, and exercises that promote independence in self-care, play, and academic duties.

3.3.4 Social Skills Development

Individuals with autism benefit from social skills training because it helps them build social competence and navigate social interactions more efficiently. These programs emphasize the importance of social cues, perspective-taking, conversational skills, and friendship-building tactics. Structured exercises, role-playing, and group therapy sessions are frequently used in social skills training to provide opportunities for developing social skills in a supportive atmosphere.

3.3.5 Cognitive-Behavioral Therapy (CBT)

Cognitive-Behavioral Therapy (CBT) is a treatment method that assists people with autism in understanding and managing their thoughts, feelings, and behaviors. CBT methods address anxiety, depression, repetitive habits, and emotional control issues. Individuals develop coping methods, problem-solving abilities, and techniques to manage stress and anxiety by identifying maladaptive patterns of thinking and behavior.

3.3.6 Sensory Integration Therapy (SIT)

Sensory integration treatment focuses on resolving sensory processing issues that are typical in people with autism. This therapy seeks to improve sensory control and integration, allowing people to respond to sensory input and engage in daily activities more effectively. Sensory integration treatment may include particular sensory activities, environmental adjustments, and self-regulation skills.

3.3.7 Parent Education and Support

Parent training and support programs are critical to empowering families with autistic children. These programs educate parents on how to support their child's development, manage challenging behaviors, and foster successful communication. Parent training may include themes such as behavioral control tactics, communication skills, and advocating for the needs of their kid.

Each autistic person may benefit from a unique combination of therapies, and treatments tailored to their strengths, problems, and requirements. When creating and implementing interventions, it is critical to consider the individual's age, developmental level, and preferences. We can assist people with autism to attain their full potential and live fulfilled lives by providing comprehensive and supportive therapies.

Sensitivity and Autism

Autism is frequently related to hypersensitivity to sensory stimuli or abnormal responses to sensory stimuli. Autism patients may have sensory sensitivities or sensory processing impairments, which can have a substantial influence on their everyday lives. Autism sensory sensitivities can emerge in a variety of ways and across multiple sensory modalities, including sight, hearing, touch, taste, and smell. Understanding and managing these sensitivities is critical for building supportive environments and fostering autism-related well-being.

Hypersensitivity is a prevalent sensory sensitivity in autism, in which individuals show an excessive response to sensory stimulation. They may be overwhelmed by loud noises or bright lights, for example, and find them uncomfortable or disturbing. Everyday sounds that others may find pleasant, such as the hum of a fluorescent light or road noise, can be quite irritating for those with autism. Similarly, some textures or garment materials may cause discomfort or irritation, which can result in aversions or meltdowns.

On the other hand, some people with autism may have hyposensitivity, which means they are less sensitive to some sensory signals. They may seek out extreme sensory experiences or participate in repetitive sensory-stimulating actions. For example, they may seek deep pressure by firmly clutching themselves or spinning in circles to feel movement.

Sensory sensitivities can have a significant influence on individuals with autism in a variety of settings. A busy shopping mall or crowded classroom, for example, with various sources of sensory input, can soon become overpowering and lead to sensory overload. Sensory sensitivity can occur, individuals with autism may struggle to filter out unnecessary sensory information and focus on the conversation or social cues, which can have an impact on social relationships.

Understanding and addressing sensory sensitivities is critical for building autism-friendly surroundings.

Some helpful strategies include:

Sensory-friendly environments: Creating locations that decrease sensory distractions, such as offering quiet areas or utilizing natural lighting, can aid in the reduction of sensory overload.

Sensory breaks: Giving individuals with autism regular pauses or time-outs in a quiet and relaxing environment might help them control their sensory experiences and recharge.

Sensory tools and supports: Offering sensory aids such as noise-canceling headphones, fidget toys, or weighted blankets can help people manage their sensory sensitivities and self-regulation.

Individualized approaches: Recognizing that each autistic person is unique, it is critical to adjust methods and accommodations to meet the individual needs of people with sensory sensitivities.

Working with professionals: Collaborating with occupational therapists or sensory integration specialists can provide significant insights and guidance in dealing with sensory sensitivities.

We can establish inclusive and supportive environments for people with autism by recognizing and addressing sensory sensitivities. Sensory sensitivities are an important aspect of the autism experience, and by understanding and addressing them, we can create a more inclusive and sensory-friendly world for all.

Menstruation and Autism

Autism and menstruation are an essential, yet frequently disregarded, problem that deserves to be addressed and understood. Menstruation, the monthly cycle experienced by people born feminine, can create specific issues for people on the autistic spectrum. Autism and menstruation are linked by sensory sensitivity, communication and social comprehension issues, and the need for specific care and instruction.

Sensory sensitivities are an important factor to consider. Because many autistic people have heightened sensory sensitivity, the sensory experiences connected with menstruation can be overpowering or painful. Sensory sensitivities can cause discomfort when wearing pads or tampons due to increased sensitivity to touch, sound, smell, and texture. Menstrual sensitivity or changes in body feelings might create anxiety or pain.

Communication and social knowledge can also help people with autism through menstruation. Many people with autism struggle to recognize and interpret social cues, nonverbal communication, and intellectual concepts. Menstruation, personal hygiene, and other related issues may necessitate clear explanations, visual assistance, and social stories to assure comprehension. Supportive environments that encourage open communication and provide clear and age-appropriate information are critical in addressing the special needs and queries of menstruating individuals with autism.

The executive functioning difficulties that are frequently associated with autism, including organization, planning, and time management, can have an impact on menstruation management. Keeping track of cycles, changing pads or tampons regularly, and maintaining personal hygiene routines might be more difficult for people with autism.

Developing methods and visual aids, such as calendars or reminders, can help to promote independence and self-care during menstruation.

Individuals with autism require adequate assistance and instruction about menstruation from their parents, carers, and educators. This could include educating people in advance about the physical and emotional changes that come with puberty and menstruation. Visual supports, social narratives, and regular routines can all help to promote comprehension, reduce anxiety, and promote independence in menstrual hygiene management.

Furthermore, addressing the unique requirements of autistic women during menstruation necessitates a comprehensive and specialized strategy. Involving healthcare practitioners, educators, and support networks in designing individualized solutions and accommodations that correspond with the individual's strengths, problems, and sensory preferences is critical. Addressing any concerns, controlling sensory sensitivities, and supporting general well-being during menstruation is critical for professionals, families, and persons with autism.

Overall, understanding the relationship between autism and menstruation is critical for providing proper assistance and education. We can empower individuals with autism to navigate menstruation with dignity, comfort, and confidence by increasing understanding, creating supportive surroundings, and providing individualized techniques. We can guarantee that menstruation is treated in a way that respects the specific needs and experiences of those on the autistic spectrum through open communication, empathy, and inclusive practices.

Conclusion

Creating a Better Future

We have gone on a journey to investigate the diverse world of autism spectrum disorder (ASD) in this book. We have investigated numerous facets of autism, from its definition and historical viewpoints to recognizing its various manifestations. We investigated the complex interplay of genetic and environmental variables and their impact on neurodevelopment. We've talked about the necessity of early detection and diagnosis, as well as the hurdles and tools available to help with prompt action. We've looked at the communication difficulties that people with autism face, as well as the solutions that can assist bridge those gaps. Furthermore, we have identified supporting interventions and therapies that enable people with autism and their families to maximize their potential and pave the path for a more promising future.

Throughout this journey, we have learned to appreciate each person on the autism spectrum for their uniqueness and personality. Autism is a rich fabric of various abilities, problems, and viewpoints, not a single thing. We've seen the tenacity and resolve of people with autism, their families, and the professionals who work relentlessly to help them.

While there is still much to learn and find about autism, our understanding of it has grown enormously over time. We have seen a shift away from considering autism as a disorder and toward acknowledging the talents and abilities that people with autism possess. We have transitioned from a deficit-based strategy to a more inclusive and strengths-based approach that recognizes and promotes neurodiversity.

It is critical to underline that acceptance, support, and inclusion are the foundations of creating a society that accepts people with autism. As we come to the end of this book, let us take the knowledge and insights we've received and apply them in our communities, schools, companies, and homes.

We can create a society where people with autism are appreciated for their unique talents and given the chances, they deserve by cultivating an environment of empathy, understanding, and acceptance. Let us work together to create a future in which people with autism thrive, grow, and leave an impact on the world.

May this book serve as a guide, an inspiration, and a catalyst for good change in the lives of people with autism and their families. As we continue on this path, keep in mind that with compassion, education, and teamwork, we can truly cultivate a brighter future for everybody.

Things to pray for on Autism Sunday

Quality of life

An end to bullying

Lifespan services

Safety from abuse

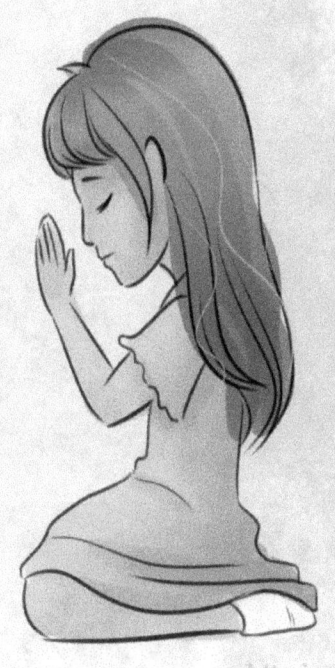

MissLunaRose

Kindness

Friendship

Understanding

Acceptance

www.ingramcontent.com/pod-product-compliance
Lightning Source LLC
Chambersburg PA
CBHW080908220526
45466CB00011BA/3503